A TO Z OF SEXUALITY

VOL. 1

25+ TYPES OF SEXUALITY

BASED ON A COMPREHENSIVE STUDY IN SEX-
POSITIVE SOCIOLOGY

BY: AIREN WILLIAMS

ISBN: 978-0-9850263-4-9

This Book Is For Everyone.

Introduction

The history of sex education is riddled with un-inclusive banter and speculation. After 21 centuries, the human race is still searching for answers about sexuality. Labels can't harness the complexity of expression, but they are tools. From birth to death, identity continues to evolve. Over a lifetime humans change physically, mentally, spiritually, emotionally and sexually.

Is love blind?

Love is more than an emotion. It is a living spirit, like oxygen it is something we need. It is something that we share with ourselves and one another. It's about perspective. How we love is how we relate to the world. It explains how we live our lives and why. It is a factor that describes how we express ourselves, how we treat other people. When you publicly or privately discuss sexuality it gets deep. Love is often perceived as light, effortless and unplanned. On the same note, love can be confusing and risky. Sexuality could be seen in a similar manner. However, modern society separates the two. Sexuality and love are not interchangeable, but studying these experiences will create a new understanding of self.

Sexuality is your sexual and sensual personality. Sexuality is a part of human identity. Denying this part of the human experience hinders our ability to reach self-actualization.   What do you like? What turns you on? What turns you off? Semi-romantic or Grey? We will look at them today. A to Z OF SEXUALITY.

Sex Geek Bonus Words

The following terms are good to know before diving into this guide through sexuality.

Human Sexuality- the way people experience and express themselves sexually. This includes but is not limited to biological, erotic, physical, emotional, social, or spiritual feelings and behaviors.

Sexual Identity- the way one thinks of oneself in terms of to whom one is romantically and/or sexually attracted. This umbrella term also refers to an individuals sexual orientation identity, biological sex, gender identity, social sex-role and sexual orientation are the four components of sexual identity.

Sexual Orientation Identity- when people identify or dis-identify with a sexual orientation or choose not to

identify with a sexual orientation.

Gender- the attitudes, behaviors,

norms and roles that a society or culture

associates with individual's sex.

Sex- sexual activity, including

specifically sexual intercourse that

involves consent.

Sexual Preference- The direction of a

person's sexual interest towards people

of the opposite sex, same sex, or both

sexes.

Sexual Attraction- an attraction

based on the basis of sexual desire.

Romantic Attraction- an attraction

that makes people desire romantic

contact.

Remember, This Book Is For Everyone.

A

Agnosexual- someone who is

undecided about their sexuality, or

someone who may have experienced

attraction to a certain gender once or a

few times but is unsure whether or not

they have a preference.

Allosexual- people who **DO** experience

sexual attraction and is used to

differentiate from people who are

asexual. Does not refer to attraction to gender. They experience sexual attraction. An allosexual can be gay, bisexual, straight, lesbian etc.

Androsexual- people who experience sexual feelings towards masculinity in general.

Asexual- people who, experience little to no interest in sexual activity

Aromantic- someone who experiences

little or no romantic attraction

regardless of sex or gender.

Autosexual- a person who is sexually

attracted to themselves.

Autoromatic- someone who is

romantically attracted to themselves.

The relationship with self is romantic

and not solely sexual or sexual at all.

B

Bicurios- a person who is questioning or exploring bisexuality. A curiosity that is romantic or sexual.

Bisexual- people who are attracted to men and women. People who are romantically or sexually attracted to more than one gender.

Biromantic- those who experience romantic attraction but not sexual attraction

D

Demiromantic- a person who can only

form romantic connections with

someone once an emotional connection

has been made. They do not experience

"love at first sight" or on sight

attraction.

Demisexual- a person that only feels

sexual attraction to someone when they

have an emotional bond with the person.

"Demi" means half- which can refer to

being halfway between sexual and

asexual. A type of gray sexuality.

E

Ecosexual- a fetish for nature and naturally occurring objects or areas, such as oceans or forests.

G

Gray sexuality- the space between sexuality and asexuality. A person experiences only a very limited amount of sexual feeling.

H

Heterosexual- a person who experiences sexual attraction to someone of an opposing gender. This typically refers to attraction between males and females.

Hobosexual- a slang term used to describe individuals who are only attracted to and aroused by people who can provide a place to stay. This is a term often used to describe men who sexually satisfy their partners for

residency convenience.

Homosexual- a person who

experiences sexual attraction to people

of the same gender. This typically refers

to attraction of men to men or women to

women.

Hypersexuality- a sexual condition

that causes one to experience much

more sexual desire than the average

person. Hypersexuals are not necessarily

sex addicts, but they constantly

experience arousal.

O

Object sexuality- people who experience sexual attraction to inanimate objects, but their lust is directed towards one or two specific objects, such as one specific chair, or in the case of one objectum sexual woman, the Eiffel Tower. Objectum sexuals typically feel a romantic connection to their chosen object as well.

Omniromantic- A person who can experience feelings of romantic love for all genders and sexualities.

Omnisexual- someone who can experience sexual attraction to those of every gender and sexuality type.

P

Pansexual- someone who feels sexual attraction to all types of people, regardless of gender or sexuality.

Polyamory- many lovers. The practice of having many multiple romantic or sexual relationships at one time. Polyamorous people tend to need sexual interactions with multiple people in order to achieve sexual happiness.

Polygamy- the practice of being

married to more than one person at a

time.

Polyromantic- someone who is

romantically attracted to several but not

all, genders or sexualities.

Polysexual- someone who is sexually

attracted to several, but not all, genders

or sexuality.

Polyunsaturated- a polyamorous

person currently seeking new sexual or

romantic relationships.

Pomoromantic- a person who

experiences romantic attraction, but

does not wish to label or define their

feelings in a conventional way.

Psychosexual- related to the mental,

emotional, or behavioral aspects of

sexuality or sexual activity.

Q

Queer- a general term for anyone
whose sexuality or gender falls outside
the "norm".

Questioning- someone who is unsure
of their sexuality, sexual preferences or
gender.

S

Sapiosexual- a type of sexuality where sexual attraction is based solely on intelligence. A sapiosexual is not blind to physicality. Physical attraction is not a deciding factor in sexual attraction.

"Nymphobraniacs" slang term.

T

Trisexual- a person who is open to
trying any kind of sexual activity. Also
called trysexual.

THIS CONCLUDES
A to Z Of SEXUALITY
VOL. 1 - 25+ Types of Sexuality

Thank you so much for reading. Be on
the lookout for the next volume. Until
then... keep this sex-positive educational
energy going!

COMMUNICATIONZ.COM

ACKNOWLEDGMENTS

This Guide through sexuality would not

be possible without the support and

mentorship that Marie Antoinette

Tichler provided. The world will change

when "Coochies Cummunicate".

References

Carrerra, M. *Sex: The Facts, the Acts, and Your Feelings.* Crown Publishers, New York. 1981.

Döring N, Mohseni MR, Walter R. *Design, Use, and Effects of Sex Dolls and Sex Robots: Scoping Review.* Journal of Medical Internet Research. 2020.

Editors of Cleis Press. *The Cleis Press Sextionary.* Cleis Press, New Jersey. 2017.

Gleik, James. *Faster: The Acceleration of Just About Everything.* Vintage Books, New York. 1999.

Gunter, Jen. *The Vagina Bible: The Vulva and the Vagina — separating the myth from the medicine.* Kensington Publishing Corp, New York. 2019.

Helman, J., & LoPiccolo, J. *Becoming Orgasmic: A Sexual and personal growth program for Women.* A Fireside Book, New York. 1988.

Morris, D. *Bodywatching: A field guide to the human species.* Crown Publishers, New York. 2002.

Navarro, Joe. *The Dictionary of Body Language; Afield Guide to Human Behavior.* Joe Navarro, New York. 2018.

Spitz, A. *The Penis Book.* Rodale Books,

Pennsylvania. 2018.

READING NOTES:

www.ingramcontent.com/pod-product-compliance
Lightning Source LLC
Chambersburg PA
CBHW022136280326
41933CB00007B/712